Slaying the Work Comp Dragon

California Workers' Compensation Acupuncture

and

The Acupuncture Expert Witness

I0483006

By

Eric M. Cachia, L.Ac.

Slaying the Work Comp Dragon
Eric M. Cachia
Kainoa Publishing Company
Santa Ana, CA 92705 USA

Copyright © 2014 Eric M. Cachia
ISBN-13:978-1497514195
ISBN-10:1497514193

Have mercy upon me,
O Lord; for I am weak:
O Lord, heal me;
for my bones are vexed.

Psalm 6:2

Dedication

To my Mother and Father

Table of Contents

Part 1

Chapter I. History of Acupuncture in California

Chapter II. History of California Workers' Compensation

Chapter III. The 2012 Workers Compensation Reform SB 863

Chapter IV. Applicant Claim Process

Chapter V. Medical Provider Network-MPN

Chapter VI. Request for Authorization and Appeal Writing

Chapter VII. Acupuncture Rehabilitation

Part 2

Chapter VIII. Acupuncture Expert Witness

Chapter XI. Conclusion

Appendix: Forms

Endnotes

Preface

Workers' compensation has helped acupuncture accelerate into main stream medicine at light speed. Acupuncture has come from antiquity to the front lines of modern health care helping injured workers return to work faster and with a minimum of side effects if any at all. Workers' compensation has helped the acupuncture profession to gain structure and purpose by providing a systematic protocol driven by a multitude of forms and questionnaires. When a practitioner first enters this complicated system it can be daunting if not a frightening and paralyzing experience for sure. Being a sound practitioner is only the beginning of several prerequisites needed to engage in this challenging yet rewarding field.

The acupuncture community has pleaded with mainstream medicine for decades to be given a chance to prove its efficacy and it has always been met with deaf ears. Mainstream medicine has always shunned acupuncture because it lacked randomized, double blind, placebo controlled trials required by the paradigm of evidence based medicine. Thanks to a few medical universities who have taken on the task to study acupuncture and present results; acupuncture is slowly proving itself. Acupuncture is now included in the California Medical Treatment Utilization Schedule (MTUS), Title 8 California Code of Regulations §9792.24.1., the American College of Occupational and Environmental practice guidelines (ACOEM), and the Official Disability Guidelines (ODG). Acupuncture is included in the California official medical fee schedule (OMFS) and included are CPT codes for acupuncture, electro-acupuncture, infrared light therapy, moxibustion, cupping, electric stimulation and a few other codes to be discussed later in this book.

The purpose of this book is to help synthesize the complexities of the constantly morphing California workers' compensation system into a palatable format so that you can begin immediately adding this dimension to your practice. It is my sincerest desire that this book will help you take your practice to the next level and enable you to begin slaying the work comp dragon.

~Eric Cachia, L.Ac.~

Part 1

Workers' Compensation Acupuncture

Chapter I

History of California Acupuncture

Acupuncture has been transformed significantly through the past several decades and the history of California acupuncture is a good place to begin to better understand where it is today.

"Before acupuncture became regulated in California, it was not uncommon for acupuncturists to be arrested and prosecuted for engaging in the practice of acupuncture. These practitioners and their patients organized and advocated for regulation to provide protection for people practicing acupuncture.

The Board of Medical Examiners began regulating acupuncture in 1972 pursuant to provisions which authorized the practice of acupuncture under the supervision of licensed physicians as part of acupuncture research in medical schools. The provisions relating to the regulation of acupuncture were amended to allow acupuncture research to be conducted under the guidance of medical schools, and $150,000 was appropriated to fund acupuncture research projects.

On July 12, 1975, the governor signed a bill that took effect immediately, creating the Acupuncture Advisory Committee. From 1975 until 1982 it was the Advisory Committee to the Division of Allied Health Professions of the Medical Board of California.

The new law authorized the practice of acupuncture, but only upon the prior diagnosis and/or referral by a physician, dentist, podiatrist or chiropractor. Consequently, prosecutions of acupuncturists, who had been arrested simply for practicing, were ordered dismissed. The law required acupuncturists to be certified, to be at least eighteen years old and of good moral character. It also required them to complete an approved acupuncture course or have two years of experience, and pass an examination administered by the then Committee.

In 1978, AB 1291 (Torres) essentially established acupuncturists as "primary health care providers" (B&P Code, section 4926) by eliminating the requirement for "prior diagnosis or referral" by a doctor, dentist, podiatrist or chiropractor; and AB 2424 (Keysor) authorized Medi-Cal payments for acupuncture treatment. Legislation was passed which established acupuncture as a certified health care profession. Certification was obtained upon successful completion of a competency examination. Also, in 1978, legislation was passed (SB 1106 (Song)) that added four public members to the Acupuncture Advisory Committee. It also clarified that the Division of Allied Health Professions (DAHP) within the Board of Medical Quality Assurance had the authority to enforce acupuncture laws; was directed to establish training standards; and was authorized to establish apprentice programs and continuing education requirements for acupuncturists. (B&P Code sections 4927, 4928, 4940 and 4945)].

In 1980, the Acupuncture Advisory Committee was abolished and replaced with the Acupuncture Examining Committee within the Division of Allied Health Professions. This allowed the Committee to have more autonomous authority; expanded acupuncturists' scope of practice to include electroacupuncture, cupping and moxibustion; and clarified that oriental massage; breathing techniques, exercise and herbs for nutrition were within the authorized practice of an acupuncturist. Fees collected from acupuncturists were no longer to be deposited into the Board of Medical Quality Assurance Fund, but into the Acupuncture Examining Committee Fund (B&P Code sections 4933 & 4937).

Legislation that passed in 1988, included acupuncturists as "physicians" only in the Workers' Compensation system for purposes of treating injured workers. The bill permitted acupuncturists to treat workplace injuries without first obtaining a referral, but limited the role of acupuncturists by not authorizing them to evaluate disability. The bill went into effect in 1989 with a four-year sunset clause. AB 400 (Chapter 824, Statutes of 1992) extended the inclusion of acupuncturists as "physicians" in the Workers' Compensation system until December 1996 and AB 1002 (Chapter 26, Statutes of 1996) further extended the inclusion of acupuncturists as "physicians" in the Workers' Compensation system until January 1, 1999. Legislation passed in 1997 (Chapter 98, Statutes of 1997) deleting the 1999 sunset date on the Workers' Compensation system.

The name of the committee was changed from "Acupuncture Examining Committee" to "Acupuncture Committee" effective January 1, 1990 (Chapter 1249, Statutes of 1989). This legislation further provided that, until January 1, 1995, the California Acupuncture Licensing Examination (CALE) would be developed and administered by an independent consultant, which was later extended to June of 2000. In September 1998 legislation was passed changing the "Acupuncture Committee" to "Acupuncture Board" to become effective January 1, 1999. The board was sunrisen until June of 2002, and the composition of the board was changed from 11 to 9 members as a result of this legislation.

In late 1999, legislation was passed (Chapter 67 (SB 1105) that eliminated the clinical portion of the examination and required that the Office of Examination Resources of the Department of Consumer Affairs develop the written examination.

The Current Acupuncture Board

As a result of legislation passed in 2005 (Chapter 659, Statutes of 2005), the board is currently comprised of seven members - four public members and three licensed acupuncturists. The Legislature has mandated that the acupuncture members of the board must represent a cross-section of the cultural backgrounds of the licensed members of the profession.

The Acupuncture Board is now an autonomous body under the umbrella of the Department of Consumer Affairs, which licenses and regulates acupuncturists in California. Pursuant to Business and Professions Code section 4925 et seq., the board administers an examination that tests an applicant's ability, competency, and knowledge in the practice of an acupuncturist; issues licenses to qualified practitioners; approves and monitors students in tutorial programs; approves acupuncture schools and continuing education providers and courses; and enforces the Acupuncture Licensure Act. The board is authorized to adopt regulations, which appear in Division 13.7, Title 16 of the California Code of Regulations".[i]

Chapter II

History of California Workers' Compensation

In 1913 the Legislature passed the Boynton Act which became effective in 1914. The Act changed workers' compensation to a compulsory program that strengthened the powers of the Industrial Accident Commission (the predecessor of DWC) to administer this program, prescribed safety regulations, among other things.

Below is the chronology of events that have molded the Workers Compensation law. Portions of the chronology are taken from the State Compensation Insurance Fund website[ii]:

Early History

1911 - Employers seek protection from injury-related litigation, and workers seek assurance of financial support while recovering from work-related injuries. As a result, reformers adopt the Roseberry Act, a voluntary workers' compensation plan. But few employers opt into the system, leading to calls for stronger laws.

1913 - The Legislature passes the Boynton Act, which creates a no-fault workers' compensation system and mandates that all employers (with a few exceptions) provide such coverage for their employees. Among its many provisions, the Act establishes a "minimum rate" law to ensure that premiums charged will be sufficient to provide financial stability for the system.

1914 - State Compensation Insurance Fund, established by the Boynton Act, opens its doors at 525 Market Street in San Francisco. Its mission is to provide an available market for workers' compensation insurance at fair rates, and to serve as a model for all carriers. In accordance with the Boynton Act, State Fund provides coverage at cost while remaining self-supporting. Though the Act appropriates $100,000 to launch the organization, State Fund never uses any of that seed money. Nevertheless, State Fund finishes its first year with $547,161.24 in premium.

Modern History:

1989 - The Legislature adopts reforms designed to reduce medical and legal expenses.

1993 - Governor Pete Wilson signs a new round of reforms to reduce costs and curb abuse of workers' compensation. The legislation repeals the minimum-rate law, effective in 1995. The new "open rating" plan sets off a period of intense competition among private insurers. While other carriers slash rates to below cost to win increased market share, State Fund maintains adequate rates. As a result, many thousands of employers leave State Fund to obtain lower-priced policies from private carriers.

1996 - As part of his Competitive Government Initiative, Governor Wilson commissions a consulting actuary firm to study the feasibility of "privatizing" State Fund. The business community roundly denounces privatization, and the governor abandons the proposal.

2003 - As result of the severe under pricing since 1995 spurred by open rating, 28 private carriers have either suffered insolvency or have stopped writing workers' compensation policies in California. Fulfilling its constitutional mandate to provide an available market, State Fund writes policies for many thousands of employers unable to find coverage elsewhere.

2005 - State Fund establishes an enhanced Medical Provider Network (MPN) to comply with 2004 reform provisions. New MPN is designed to enhance access to medical treatment for injured workers and reduce medical treatment costs for employers. Over 10,000 health care providers at 10,000 facilities become part of MPN.

2006 - Competition returns to California's workers' comp market as savings from 2004 reform materialize. State Fund begins to shed market share, increases reserves and surplus and strengthens financial position.

2007 – Board of Directors appoints first State Fund President and CEO from private industry.

California Department of Insurance (CDI) reviews State Fund operations and provides recommendations. State Fund begins transformative change as it strengthens corporate governance and focuses on improving transparency and accountability within the organization.

2008 – Legislature passes State Fund governance laws that expand the Board of Directors, creates additional exempt executive positions and makes State Fund subject to California Public Records and Bagley-Keene Opening Meeting Acts.

2009 – Gov. Arnold Schwarzenegger taps four new members and reappoints a sitting member to the 11-person State Fund Board of Directors.

2010 – The Board appoints Tom Rowe as State Fund President, CEO and member of the Executive Committee on August 2, 2010.

2012 – SB 863, major workers' compensation reform to raise permanent disability benefits and cost savings to the system, signed by Governor Brown.

2013 – Department of Workers' Compensation adopts Medicare fee schedule.

Chapter III

The 2012 Workers Compensation Reform SB 863

Senate Bill 863 (SB 863) was the product of months of negotiations between representatives of labor unions and employers who historically came together to work on a comprehensive workers' compensation reform package. Everything in SB 863 was negotiated and agreed on by those parties.

The negotiators started with two guiding principles. First, that permanent disability benefits paid to injured workers to compensate them for the lasting effects of work-related injuries were too low and had to be increased. The second principle was that the costs associated with providing medical treatment and benefits to injured workers and administering workers' compensation claims had begun to rise significantly. If costs were permitted to continue to rise, employers would be faced with increases in their workers' compensation insurance rates, which would add additional financial stress to many businesses.

Labor and management agreed that in order for benefits to be increased, costs would have to be decreased where possible. They also agreed that where possible, the workers' compensation process should be made more efficient.

Implementation of the changes brought about by the bill will be overseen by teams from both the California Department of Industrial Relations (DIR) and the Division of Workers' Compensation (DWC).

The following are some of the highlights of the bill:

Changes in Permanent Disability

Both the minimum and maximum weekly benefit amounts have been increased, with the increases being phased in over a two year period. At the end of those two years, the maximum weekly permanent disability rate will rise to $290.

How permanent disability ratings are calculated has also been changed. The current rating formula includes a modifier of between 1.1 and 1.4, depending on the body part that is injured. The modifier is intended to take into account the injured workers' diminished future earning capacity, if any, as a result of his or her injury. For injuries that occur on or after Jan. 1, 2013, the rating formula will no longer include the "future earning capacity modifier." Instead, all injuries will be adjusted by a factor of 1.4.

Under the current rating system, there are also modifiers based on the injured worker's age at the time of the injury, and his or her occupation. Those modifiers will continue to be used, and the Administrative Director of the Division of Workers' Compensation has been authorized to develop a new schedule of occupational modifiers, to allow for more accurate consideration of today's wide range of occupations.

Currently, Labor Code Section 4662 describes circumstances in which injured workers may receive a permanent disability award of 100%. That section has not been changed by SB 863.

Add-ons for permanent disability due to sleep disorders or sexual dysfunction resulting from physical injuries, which are now permitted, will no longer be available. Additionally, permanent disability add-ons for psychiatric injuries resulting from physical injuries are limited to "catastrophic" injuries and cases in which the injured worker was either the victim of a violent crime, or witnessed a violent crime.

"Pure" psychiatric claims which do not arise as a result of physical injuries are not affected by this change. Injured workers can still receive treatment for sleep problems, sexual dysfunction and/or psych consequences of their injuries, even if permanent disability is no longer available for them.

Changes to Supplemental Job Displacement Vouchers

Under the current system, injured workers may be offered supplemental job displacement vouchers that can be used to pay for job retraining. The voucher amount is a sliding scale ranging from $4,000 to $10,000. The amount is based upon the injured worker's permanent disability rating, and it is not required to be offered until the permanent disability rating has been finally determined, either by way of an award by the Workers' Compensation Appeals Board (WCAB), or by a settlement agreement between the injured worker and his or her employer.

As a result of SB 863, the voucher amount will be fixed at $6,000 for all qualifying injured workers, and it is to be offered when the injured worker reaches permanent and stationary status and the treating doctor reports on work abilities and limitations resulting from the injury.

Creation of "Return to Work Fund"

SB 863 also establishes a $120 million per year "Return-to-Work Fund," to be established and administered by the DIR. Payments from the fund will be available to injured workers whose permanent disability ratings are disproportionately low in comparison to their wage loss. Eligibility for the benefits and the specifics of how the fund will be administered will be based on research to be performed by the DIR in consultation with the Commission on Health, Safety and Workers' Compensation (CHSWC).

Injured workers will be able to appeal decisions regarding Return to Work Fund eligibility or the amount to be paid out will be to the trial-level WCAB.

Introduction of Independent Medical Review

Another significant change is in how medical treatment disputes will be resolved. As of Jan. 1, 2013 for injuries occurring on or after that date, and as of July 1, 2013 for all dates of injury, Independent Medical Review (IMR) will be used to decide disputes regarding medical treatment in workers' compensation cases.

Under the current system, it typically takes nine to 12 months to resolve a dispute over the treatment needed for an injury. The process requires: (1) negotiating over selection of an agreed medical evaluator, (2) obtaining a panel, or list, of state-certified medical evaluators if agreement cannot be reached, (3) negotiating over the selection of the state-certified medical evaluator, (4) making an appointment, (5) awaiting the examination, (6) awaiting the evaluator's report, and then if the parties still disagree, (7) awaiting a hearing with a workers' compensation judge and (8) awaiting the judge's decision on the recommended treatment. In many cases, the treating physician may also rebut or request clarification from the medical evaluator, and the medical evaluator may be required to follow up with supplemental reports or answer questions in a deposition.

SB 863 replaces those eight steps with an IMR process similar to group health that takes approximately 40 (or fewer) days to arrive at a determination so that the appropriate treatment can be obtained.

IMR can only be requested by an injured worker following a denial, modification, or delay of a treatment request through the utilization review (UR) process. Employers and insurance carriers cannot request review of treatment authorizations.

An injured worker can be assisted by an attorney or by his or her treating physician in the IMR process.

There is a right to appeal an IMR determination, to the trial level WCAB, on the basis of fraud, conflict of interest, or mistake of fact. The reviewer's underlying medical decision-making, however, cannot be overturned by a judge. The remedy, if an appeal is granted, is referral to a different reviewer for another review.

IMR will not be available in cases in which there is a dispute over anything other than the medical necessity of a particular treatment requested by the injured worker's physician (such as cases where the injury itself is in dispute).

Improving Medical Provider Networks

Medical Provider Networks (MPNs) have been criticized for including doctors who are no longer practicing, do not accept workers' compensation patients, or are otherwise unavailable to injured workers. Injured workers have also expressed frustration at not being able to obtain care in specialty areas, and doctors not being available within reasonable time frames.

SB 863 addresses these issues in several ways. First, the current requirement that 25% of doctors within an MPN practice in areas other than occupational medicine has been removed. Also, doctors are required to affirmatively confirm their participation in a network.

Networks will also be required to provide medical access assistants who will be available to injured workers to assist them in locating appropriate doctors within the network.

SB 863 also provides for better monitoring of MPNs by the DWC through continuous and random reviews, and authority to impose penalties less severe than revocation to address access problems.

Additionally, disputes about whether or not an injured worker is subject to an MPN will now have to be resolved as soon as they arise, rather than being held over to the end of a claim. Treatment obtained from a non-network provider, without either authorization from the employer or insurance carrier or a workers' compensation judge's order permitting outside of network treatment, will not have to be paid for by the employer or carrier. If unauthorized treatment is unsuccessful, and results in a worsening of the injured worker's condition, or a need for additional treatment, the employer/carrier will have no obligation to pay for that, either.

Similarly, reports issued by unauthorized non-network providers cannot be the sole basis for an award of compensation by a workers' compensation judge. Those reports must be reviewed and commented on by the authorized network provider and any qualified medical evaluator (QME) or agreed medical evaluator (AME).

Introduction of Independent Medical Review

SB 863 creates an In Independent Bill Review (IBR) process to resolve disputes regarding the amount to be paid to doctors.

IBR will not apply to disputes about treatment authorization (those will go through IMR), cases where the injury itself is in dispute, or where there is a dispute about whether or not the provider is authorized to treat the injured worker.

There are also new requirements regarding how billing is to be submitted, and how employers or carriers communicate their payment decisions to providers.

Changes regarding liens

There are also changes regarding liens filed against an injured workers' claim, for medical treatment and other services provided in connection with the claim, but not paid for by the employer or insurance carrier.

A filing fee of $150 will now be required for all liens filed after Jan. 1, 2013, and a $100 activation fee will be required for liens filed before then, but activated for a conference or trial after Jan. 1, 2013.

There are also provisions for dismissal of liens by operation of law after Jan. 1, 2014 if no filing or activation fee has been filed, as well as an 18-month statute of limitations for filing liens for services rendered after July 1, 2013 and a 3-year statute of limitations for services provided before then. Assignments of lien claims are also now strictly limited, and are allowed only where the assignor has gone out of business.

Fee Schedule

SB 863 requires the creation of fee schedules for copy services, home health care, vocational expert fees and interpreters. The DWC will also be able to administer interpreter certification exams and post lists of certified interpreters on its web site.

The Official Medical Fee Schedule (OMFS), which governs fees paid to medical providers, will also be updated, to incorporate Medicare's Resource-Based Relative Value Scale.

Changes for Qualified and Agreed Medical Evaluators

There is a new limit of ten office locations for QMEs.

In cases in which the injured worker is represented by an attorney, there is no longer a requirement that the parties try to reach an agreement on an AME before seeking a QME panel. Additionally, in cases in which the injured worker is represented, the parties may agree to use an AME.

Changes for Self Insured Employers

Self-insured employers are required to pay deposits to help ensure that their workers' compensation liabilities will be covered. SB 863 changes the method of calculating the deposit amount, basing it now on an annual actuarial report to be issued by Dec. 31 of every year.

The bill also precludes "professional employer organizations," temporary agencies, and employee leasing organizations from being self-insured, as well as prohibiting an employer who has been illegally uninsured from becoming self-insured unless the employer receives approval from the Self-Insurers' Security Fund.

Self-insured public entities' annual reporting requirements have been strengthened, and CHSWC is now required to study the self-insured public entity program and make recommendations to improve the program. The CHSWC study is expected to be completed by mid-2014.[iii]

Chapter IV

Applicant Claim Process

There are two different attorneys at work in a workers' compensation case: The applicant attorney represents the injured worker and the defense attorney is normally retained by the insurance company of the employers business that has a policy with them. When an injured worker files a claim against the employer, he or she has the right to receive up to $10,000 in medical care under treatment guidelines while the employer decides whether to accept or deny the claim. The employer must approve that treatment within one working day of receiving the injured workers' claim form.

The Primary Treating Physician (PTP) is the doctor with the overall responsibility for treatment of injury or illness. Generally the employer selects the PTP the worker will see for the first 30 days, however, in specified conditions, the injured party may be treated by a predesignated doctor or medical group. If a doctor says treatment is still needed after 30 days, the worker may be able to switch to the doctor of their choice. Different rules apply if the employer is using a Health Care Organization (HCO) or a Medical Provider Network (MPN). A MPN is a selected network of health care providers to provide treatment to workers injured on the job. The employee should receive information from their employer if they are covered by an HCO or a MPN. They would need to contact the employer for more information. If the employer has not put up a poster describing employee rights to workers' compensation, the employee may choose their own doctor immediately.

Applicant	Defense
Employee	Employer
Applicant Attorney-Employee Worker covered by Workers' Compensation Insurance	Defense Attorney-Employer Workers' Compensation insurance carrier
Applicant Physician-PTP Primary Treating Physician	Defense Physician AME Agreed Medical Evaluator

Injured workers are entitled to receive all medical care reasonably required to cure or relieve the effects of the injury, with no deductible or co-payments by the injured worker. For dates of injury on or after Jan. 1, 2004, an injured worker is limited to 24 chiropractic and 24 physical therapy visits. *There is no limit on acupuncture so long as functional improvement can be demonstrated.*

Chapter V

Medical Provider Network
MPN

A medical provider network (MPN) is an entity or group of health care providers set up by an insurer or self-insured employer and approved by DWC's administrative director to treat workers injured on the job. Under state regulations, each MPN must include a mix of doctors specializing in work-related injuries and doctors with expertise in general areas of medicine. MPNs are required to meet access to care standards for common occupational injuries and work-related illnesses. The regulations also require MPNs to follow all medical treatment guidelines established by the DWC and allow employees a choice of provider(s) in the network after their first visit. Additionally, MPNs must offer an opportunity for second and third opinions if the injured worker disagrees with the diagnosis or treatment offered by the treating physician. If a disagreement still exists after the second and third opinion, an injured worker in the MPN may request an independent medical review (IMR). The MPN program became effective Jan. 1, 2005 and employees can be covered by an MPN once a plan has been approved by the DWC administrative director.

Injured workers have been frustrated by the delays they have encountered in obtaining effective treatment approved by the insurers. MPNs were designed to minimize these delays because insurer objections to proposed treatments in theory should be reduced because as insurers would have more confidence that MPN doctors are following appropriate medical treatment guidelines.

The system was created to ensure that injured workers have easy access to treatment and so the regulations require MPNs in urban areas to ensure that a primary care physician and a hospital for emergency care are located within a close proximity of each employee's residence or place of work. Specialists must also need to be within a reasonable driving range. Alternate standards for rural areas must be approved by the administrative director of DWC on a case-by-case basis.

The regulations provide safeguards for workers injured prior to the establishment of approved MPNs by allowing them to continue to receive treatment from their existing doctor(s) if the worker is scheduled for surgery, or the worker's condition is acute, serious and chronic or terminal.[iv]

As of the date of this printing, acupuncturists are not required to be part of the MPN. The PTP however needs to be on one or more MPN panel(s). It is very unlikely that you would be referred a patient where the PTP is not on a panel, however; if the case is denied then a case could be referred on a lien basis (this will be discussed later).

Chapter VI

Request for Authorization
and Appeal Writing

The request for authorization to treat is normally requested by the PTP on a form known as a PR-2 (check the back of the book for all forms). The PTP will likely be an orthopedist, physiatrist or interventional pain specialist. The PTP requests whatever he considers necessary to diagnose and treat the current injury sustained by the worker. This will include different types of treatment such as surgery, medications, injections, physical therapy, chiropractic, acupuncture and more.

Normally the patient will come to you authorized to treat but on many occasions they will not. If the PTP does not send you the patient authorized you will need to request authorization on yet another form. The authorization process is slow but at some point you will receive an authorization for treatment or a denial based on medical necessity. If the claim is denied altogether and you wish to treat anyways then you will need to file a lien. You will have to make a decision whether or not you are willing to wait until the case closes which could be anywhere from a few months to several years.

The authorization will come from the claims adjuster of the insurance company and dictate how many treatment visits have been granted and at times specify a period of time to complete the treatment by. It is imperative that you communicate with both the

PTP and the claims adjuster as to the progress of the patient. A simple one page SOAP note addressed to both the PTP and claims adjuster will suffice. Make sure you send one copy to each and place the original in the patients file. The report should include the patients name, the claim number, the date of injury, the diagnosis, how may treatments the patient has had; the progress and your request for additional treatments if the patient has demonstrated adequate functional improvement.

As previously stated if the claim is denied as to the cause of injury you will need to file a lien. But if the case is denied based on medical necessity then you will want to appeal the case to the adjuster. Normally you will have 30 days from the date of the denial to send an appeal to the claims adjuster. The non-certification or denial letter that is sent from the insurance company claims adjuster will cite the reasons for their denial. Don't let this intimidate you from seeking the best interest for your patient. The denial letter will tell you exactly why in their opinion the authorization has been denied. Whatever the case is you have the weight of the law to make your appeal. Section §9792.24.1 of the Acupuncture Medical Treatment Guidelines is what needs to be quoted on your appeal letter which states in part that a trial of acupuncture is medically necessary. If the authorization for treatment is denied after you have requested for additional therapy then you will need to address at least two areas of functional improvement to be successful in your appeal letter.

Chapter VII

Acupuncture Rehabilitation

Workers' compensation acupuncture is markedly different from private acupuncture practice. The workers' compensation system is a machine that runs on the foundation of a multidisciplinary clinical setting. Acupuncture school clinics allow for a significant amount of time the student can spend with the patient but in the real world clinical setting time is very limited and you will likely be treating more than one patient simultaneously. Some acupuncturists try to practice using the Oriental medicine style of treatment but in most cases this will hamper your efficiency. A medical acupuncture style is better suited to the workers' compensation acupuncture clinic.

Many cases will require the use of electric acupuncture because the main issue you will be addressing for the patient is pain. Most cases will require physical therapy and if the patient is in extreme pain then you will be very helpful to the PTP and the patient. These medical doctors on the whole are very positive in their attitude towards the efficacy of acupuncture as it aids the physical therapist to do their jobs more efficiently because the acupuncturist can diminish pain which in turn reduces guarding. Guarding is when the patient protects their injured body part by resisting the action or exercise that the physical therapist tries to employ in their rehabilitation program. Guarding is a problem as it hinders or delays the progress of the patient. The objective is to get the patient functional as soon as possible allowing for a quicker return to work.

Below is a short list of CPT codes normally used in the acupuncture treatment. The combined therapy can be no longer than one hour and each code is for 15 minutes of treatment time up to 4 codes. No more than 2 timed procedures and 2 modalities:

New Patient Exam:

99203 Detailed

99204 Comprehensive

Re Evaluation Exam:

99212 Limited

99213 Detailed

Acupuncture

97810 Acupuncture, one or more needles, without electrical stimulation, initial 15 min.

97811 Acupuncture, one or more needles, without electrical stimulation, each additional 15 minutes. With re-insertion.

Electric Acupuncture:

97813 Acupuncture, one or more needles, with electrical stimulation, initial 15 minutes.

97814 Acupuncture, one or more needles, with

electrical stimulation, each additional 15 minutes. With re-insertion.

Physical Therapy procedure:

97140 Myofascial Release

Modalities:

97026 Infrared

97014 Electric Stimulation

97802 Cupping

97803 Moxibustion

Part 2

The Acupuncture
Expert Witness

Chapter VIII

Acupuncture Expert Witness

You might be asking yourself the question why would I want to become a forensic acupuncture expert witness? There are several good reasons for wanting to become a forensic acupuncture expert witness. Let's examine a few basic reasons and benefits to engage oneself in this rewarding field of opportunity.

- I am an expert in the field acupuncture and oriental medicine.

- I can protect the public by raising the bar in the standard of care for patients.

- The profession of acupuncture and oriental medicine will enjoy a more professional image and respect by the public and other health care professionals.

- A forensic acupuncture expert can be a fulfilling profession whether on a part time or full time basis.

- I can both help protect and contribute to the profession that I have enjoyed and also provide a value added service as member of the ancient art and science of acupuncture and oriental medicine.

I am an expert in acupuncture and oriental medicine.

It's true! You have spent tortured days and nights for years memorizing acupuncture points single herbs, herbal formulas and many other treatment modalities. You have also consumed volumes of extensive medical reading material in both eastern and western medicine. You have likely studied and prepared for both your state board exam as well the national board exams. You may have even acquired a special certification or two and possibly even become board certified in specialty areas such as Orthopedics, Oriental Physical Medicine, acupuncture injection therapy or the N.A.D.A. protocol. You have expanded your knowledge by completing numerous continuing education courses to maintain your state and or national licenses and certifications respectively.

Beyond these basic competencies you have gained years of clinical experience treating a multitude of various complex health issues and in doing so have matured as a clinician to the point that you have begun to give back to the acupuncture and oriental profession by educating others in the field as a provider of continuing education or taking on a professor position at one of our approximately 50 fine acupuncture and oriental medicine institutions. Your career path may have led your practice into the med legal arenas of workers compensation and or personal injury necessitating the interaction with specialist attorneys. It's possible that you have joined one of a multiplicity of various acupuncture and oriental medicine associations to stay current in the profession as well as to help advance the acupuncture and oriental medicine profession to the next level. Perhaps you may have even sat in on a committee or been a board member on the state level or some special interest group. The sum of all these experiences sets you apart from the general public, other health care professionals, attorneys, judges and juries. Only you can provide a sound independent opinion because you are an expert in the field of acupuncture and oriental medicine.

I can protect the public by raising the bar in the standard of care for patients.

All health care professionals take a vow or oath and you normally find somewhere in these documents specific language that reads you as future licensed healthcare professional promises to "do no harm" Our profession of acupuncture and oriental medicine is no different. This is exactly why we have schools that are licensed to grant diplomas or degrees from various state boards of education and other agencies and is exactly the reason we have state licenses or certifications and other forms of minimal level competency accounting. All these various forms of check points serve to protect the public. Most states and other jurisdictions have an acupuncture act and this body of law serves to produce what is known as a minimal competency level or *standard of care* in the community.

When a violation of a state acupuncture act occurs it is the responsibility of the state board to act upon the complaint made and either resolve that complaint with a disciplinary action or a dismissal within the jurisdiction of the board or referral of the case file to the attorney general of the particular state where the allegation occurred for disposition of the case. Whether the case remains on the state board level or is referred to the states attorney the services of a forensic acupuncture expert maybe required in the form of a *statement of opinion* for further legal analysis so that either entity can proceed with the case or dispose of the matter altogether. There maybe be more work involved as a expert if a deposition and or trial is required and discussion of these various stages of litigation will be addressed in the appropriate section of this book but it should becoming more apparent that only you can provide a sound independent opinion because you are an expert and in doing so you will in part help in protecting the public by raising the bar in the *standard of care* for patients.

The profession of acupuncture and oriental medicine will enjoy a more professional image and respect by the public and other health care professionals.

The ancient art and science of acupuncture and oriental medicine has endured the test of time and continues to demonstrate itself as an efficacious form of health care but the community as a whole has struggled to be perceived as a viable component of the modern health care paradigm. There are many possible explanations for this current dilemma such as the division between the fundamentalist oriental philosophy of acupuncturists who seek to preserve the ancient traditions and the acupuncturists who pursue the integration of the ancient traditions with modern science, techniques and technology. These differences have fostered an atmosphere of discontent in various factions within the acupuncture and oriental medicine community. Also, the acupuncture and oriental medicine community has not been able to come together to form a strong uniform coalition such as the American Medical Association or American Chiropractic Association.

These and other issues have slowed the process in advancement of acceptance in western thinking and perception. Whatever the explanation is this may have affected the ability of acupuncture and oriental medicine to climb up the proverbial medical totem pole. As acupuncture continues to maneuver its way into a solidified body of health care practitioners you as an expert can contribute to the positive perception of the community with this noble service. Serving as an expert witness helps the governing bodies to separate the public from incompetent or criminal activity committed by a few practitioners. This rewarding function as an expert will in some way aid the profession of acupuncture and oriental medicine to enjoy a more professional image and respect by the public and other health care professionals.

Being a forensic acupuncture expert can be a fulfilling profession whether part time or full time.

There are several benefits to becoming a forensic acupuncture expert which can be either performed on either a part time or full time capacity. A Curriculum Vitae complete with some or all of the career fulfillment mentioned previously with the added expert witness designation is sure to catch the eye of any interested party. Also, becoming an expert witness can be a very lucrative profession as expert witnesses command a handsome salary if done on a regular basis and the expert witness fees are set according to the standard fees in the community being served. Expert witnesses enjoy a certain level of respect within and outside the area of expertise that is being served by the expert witness.

Another benefit is that serving as an expert witness can supplement your current clinical practice earnings and or transition you to a consultant as you approach the end of your clinical career because many Oriental medicine practitioners find it difficult to maintain a full time practice and this is a wonderful use of any down time you have in your current practice.

You will also enjoy the process of preparing yourself to become an expert witness. There are many courses that you can take to help you in your journey and all while earning a certification as an expert. Many of these courses can be found in the extension university of either the UC or State systems in California. If you are not in California then you will want to check the education system in your particular state. Forensic organizations also have courses and seminars offered to help to help you polish your skills. You may even want to check with your local bar association as they are often an excellent resource for upcoming seminars and also for networking.

Whether your goal is to improve the credentials of your CV, increase revenue potential or serve the public you will find that these are just a few reasons being a forensic acupuncture expert can be a fulfilling profession whether on a part time or full time capacity.

I can both help protect and contribute to the profession that I have enjoyed and also provide a value added service as a member of the ancient art and science of acupuncture and oriental medicine.

You have spent a lot of resources both time and money to become a professionally licensed clinician. Our profession also has spanned centuries and stood the test of time. Despite all of this all it takes is a few rogue events to undo all the magic and wonder of our ancient profession. Becoming an expert in acupuncture and Oriental medicine is clearly one of the most noble of pursuits in our profession because you as an expert will be standing guard and defending our profession.

Unfortunately our profession has been a target for cases concerning moral turpitude. The State of California has even placed a formal warning on acupuncturists because there are some who have used acupuncture as a clinic front for a brothel. Sadly, these and other instances of moral turpitude have affected the public perception of our profession and now more than ever there is a need for experts to step up and make a statement of opinion as to the standard of care in the community. This will help not only to punish criminal behavior and send a warning signal to criminals but to also demonstrate to the public that we can self regulate by serving as experts.

Another way to protect and to contribute to the profession is to help with the disposition of acupuncturists that in rare events injure patients. This function serves primarily to protect the public but by doing so protects the profession. The focus here is not that of a conspiracy against the acupuncturist but to seek out the truth and construct a rehabilitation program to bring the acupuncturist back up to the minimum level of the standard of care required to practice and to prevent a recurrence of the injury.

As you can see by becoming and expert witness one can both help protect and contribute to the profession that we have enjoyed and also provide a value added service as member of the ancient art and science of acupuncture and oriental medicine.

What your job is as an expert witness and the services that are performed.

- *Investigation*. Your client (attorney) will send you all the documents to investigate and you will in turn research everything written on the particular issue and then evaluate the information collected.

- *Evaluation*. You will evaluate and submit a written report of your findings as to the merits of the case whether a standard of care or other issue.

- *Consult*. You will advise the attorney and possibly judge and or jury as to what transpired or what should be the outcome in the case.

- *Testify*. Unlikely, but you may be subpoenaed to testify in a deposition or in trial before a judge and jury. The case is most often settled out of court.

- *Writing skills*. You do need to be articulate as it is imperative that you can express your ideas in writing in such a way that a jury can understand what you are trying to convey to them.

- *Credible witness*. Emanates from your education, degree, specialty and experience. You must be perceived as objective and convincing.

Your report should appear professional and be printed on a high quality laser printer. Here is an example of an outline to write a report:

- Title and cover-Standard of Care Opinion

- Table of Contents

- Definitions

- Synopsis of Medical History

- Standard of Care

- Conclusion

- References/Attachments

The next thing you will need is a contract and fee schedule.

Below is an example of a contract and fee schedule:

Expert Witness Fees &
Acupuncture Expert Services Agreement

Litigation: $250.00 per hour for services including, but not limited to, review, research and analysis: reports, conferences, site visitation and survey where appropriate together with a review of all discovery materials and any other materials deemed necessary to reach and render an opinion in the subject litigation.

A minimum, non-refundable advance retainer fee of $2,000.00 is required. Initial work will be charged against the retainer. I am retained solely by the attorney/attorney's firm (client) and no relationship exists between the attorney's client and me. The attorney/attorney firm is solely responsible for fee payment.

Deposition: Deposition fee will be $1000.00 to be pre paid by opposing counsel on or before the date of deposition.

Trial: $2,000.00 or a full eight (8) hours for trial appearance and testimony.

Cancellation: Counsel is required to provide forty-eight (48) hour notice of cancellation of scheduled testimony or be subject to a four (4) hour cancellation fee plus any travel expenses.

Travel: Client is responsible for travel arrangements and actual expenses. Travel fees are billed at $60.00 per hour. No fees will be advanced by this office.

Invoices: All invoices are due and payable within 15 (15) days of receipt. Invoices thirty (30) days past due will be charged interest at the rate of 1.5% per month (annual rate of 18%), and will be assessed a $200.00 late fee. Invoices sixty (60) days past due will be referred for collection and all legal remedies for payment pursued.

Payment: The attorney/attorney firm is solely responsible for fee payment.

Engagement: Your signature below indicates acceptance of this binding agreement and formal engagement of John Q. Acupuncturist, L.Ac. to provide expert witness services.

Authorized Signature / Title: _____

Date: _____

Marketing Strategy

If you are inclined to become an acupuncture expert witness you will need to have a marketing strategy. You will need to make yourself visible by promoting yourself with marketing. Below are some suggestions you can use to begin an excellent marketing program. Send your CV, marketing literature and fee schedule to the following:

- *State and Local Agencies*. This will include your state Acupuncture board, Attorney General, and the District Attorney's of counties that you want to service.

- *Expert Witness Agencies*. Search the internet for expert witness agencies. Some are completely free and others charge fees. Start out with what you can afford and don't be afraid to start off with free services to see if you get some leads. Most of these directories require a CV and your fee schedule.

- *Take a seminar*. As previously stated take some forensic courses. Many localities have forensic associations.

- *Speaking engagement*. Speak at a legal seminar or education training course. This will give attorneys an opportunity to hear you as well as learn about your acupuncture expertise.

- *Word of mouth*. Inform everyone you are positioning yourself to be an expert witness.

- *Referrals*. As you gain expertise and experience you will get more referrals.

- *Email marketing*. There are email marketing companies online where you can purchase email lists by zip code. You can start out very simple and cost effective by marketing just a few zip codes.

- *Network*. Most acupuncturists will be intimidated by the thought of the litigation process let alone going inside a courtroom so there may not be a lot of competition. Inform all your colleagues, the acupuncture associations and magazines related to acupuncture that you are available for expert services.

- *Write an article*. Write about your experiences in forensics as an expert witness for acupuncture journals and other publications.

Certification courses and training

There are basically 3 different ways to improve your skills to become a highly skilled expert and therefore more marketable:

- **Online courses**. There are literally hundreds of online courses, seminars and certifications available. You will need to carefully screen out the worthless courses and seek a course that most closely relates to the acupuncture specialty which will likely be a course that focuses on the medical professional.

- **Classroom Courses**. Some universities offer a "Forensic expert certification" course. These courses are very useful because many times they simulate the real process of being an expert; e.g., narrative writing practice as well as mock deposition and trial practice.

- **Forensic association courses**. There are a number a forensic associations and they often hold topical seminars and training for both its member and non-members. Check with a local forensic entity for a listing of current courses and seminars being offered.

It should be fairly clear by now whether a career as a forensic acupuncture expert is something you would like to undertake. Being an expert witness is not for everyone especially those who are sensitive or do not find adversarial debate appealing. Whether you want to pursue this or not you have learned something new that will definitely broaden your intellectual horizon. For those of you who wish to become a forensic acupuncture expert witness I encourage you to consume as many books and publications as possible on the subject that go into specific details far beyond the outline and purpose of this book.

Chapter IX

Conclusion

This book was written based on the interest generated by acupuncturists who approached me to learn more in detail how to better integrate Workers' Compensation cases into their practice. Please review all the forms listed at the end of this book to create your own personalized forms. This particular area of acupuncture will definitely supplement and round out your practice. Also listed at the end of this book are basic protocols I have found successful in treating common maladies associated with work related injuries. Also, work as an expert witness is very valuable and you will acquire knowledge previously unknown which will make you a very well rounded clinician.

It is my hope that you have gained insight into the California Workers' Compensation System and work as a Forensic Expert Witness sufficiently that the information provided will benefit you and your practice.

Appendix

Functional Improvement

Acupuncture functional improvement language examples for Medical Necessity or Appeal. The appropriate line(s) should be selected to insert in your letter based on the body part treated.

1. Pt. presented with a 7/10 VAS pain score and after a course of acupuncture is now a 5/10.
2. Pt. complained of sleeping only 4 hours a night and after acupuncture tx is now sleeping 6 hours.
3. Pt. has reduced medications to prn after a course of acupuncture tx.
4. Pt. complained of only being able to walk for 15 minutes or less because of pain and is now able to walk 30 minutes after a course of acupuncture.
5. Pt. was unable to raise shoulder above _____ level; now able to lift arm above _____ level after a course of acupuncture tx.
6. Grip/grasp/pull was difficult prior to course of acupuncture tx.

Mental Health referral to Acupuncture

The Acupuncture Medical Treatment Guidelines set forth in this subdivision shall supersede the text in the ACOEM Practice Guidelines, Second Edition, relating to acupuncture, except for shoulder complaints, and shall address acupuncture treatment where not discussed in the ACOEM Practice Guidelines.

(A) Definitions per MTUS:

(i) "Acupuncture" is used as an option when pain medication is reduced or not tolerated, it may be used as an adjunct to physical rehabilitation and/or surgical intervention to hasten functional recovery. It is the insertion and removal of filiform needles to stimulate acupoints (acupuncture points). Needles may be inserted, manipulated, and retained for a period of time. Acupuncture can be used to reduce pain, reduce inflammation, increase blood flow, increase range of motion, decrease the side effect of medication-induced nausea, **promote relaxation in an anxious patient**, and reduce muscle spasm.

(B) Psych. Conditions that can benefit from acupuncture treatment:

Example of Psych. Services patients that can benefit from acupuncture (not limited to these conditions only): See references below
1. Generalized Anxiety disorders
2. Other conditions based on your impression if acupuncture would relax and benefit the patient

(C) Contraindications:
- Pregnancy, esp. in first trimester
- Bleeding disorders, anticoagulants, and anti-platelet drugs
- Immuno-compromised patients
- Skin infections at site of needling
- Skin disorders such as psoriasis or eczema
- Valvular heart disease

- o Patients who are going to drive or operate machinery
- o Demand pacemaker (electro-acupuncture)

(D) Suggested protocol:
- Acupuncture trial twice per week for 3 weeks thereafter re-evaluate. See MTUS guidelines.

(E) Discussion: Acupuncture releases a formulary of endorphins, enkephalins and neurotransmitters. Acupuncture causes the patient to subjectively have a sense of well-being and relaxation.

References: Authority cited: Sections 133, 4603.5, 5307.3 and 5307.27, Labor Code. Reference: Sections 77.5, 4600, 4604.5 and 5307.27, Labor Code.

Progress Report to Primary Treating Physician

[ ] Periodic Report
[ ] Change in treatment plan
[ ] Request to continue treatment
[ ] Change in patient's condition
[ ] Information request

Patient Name:_____

DOB:_____

DOI:_____

Claims
Administrator:_____

Claim
number:_____

Subjective complaints:

Objective findings:

Diagnoses:

Treatment plan:

Signature:_____Date:_____

Pain Scale

Patient Name: _____
Area of Pain: _____

Rate the severity of your pain by checking one box on the following scale.

0 1 2 3 4 5 6 7 8 9 10
No Pain Unbearable
Pain
Today's Date: _____ Initial: _____

Rate the severity of your pain by checking one box on the following scale.

0 1 2 3 4 5 6 7 8 9 10
No Pain Unbearable
Pain
Today's Date: _____ Initial: _____

Rate the severity of your pain by checking one box on the following scale.

0 1 2 3 4 5 6 7 8 9 10
No Pain Unbearable
Pain
Today's Date: _____ Initial: _____

WORKERS COMP PRE-AUTHORIZATION REQUEST

Date: _____/_____/_____   Claim#:

_____

Insurance Carrier/ UR:

_____

Patient: _____   DOI:

_____

1. Diagnosis: _____

2: Last Exam Date & Findings:

_____

Subjective:

_____ Pain: ☐Right ☐Left

☐Cervical ☐Thoracic ☐Lumbar ☐Elbow ☐Wrist ☐Shoulder ☐Hip ☐Knee ☐Ankle ☐Foot

_____ Increased pain with walking and standing

Objective:

_____ Pain with palpation to above indicated area.

_____ Swelling in above indicated area

_____ Decreased range of motion in above indicated area

_____ Pain with range of motion

3. **Recommended Services / Procedures**
    Treatment Plan:
    _____ Acupuncture treatment to affected area

    Frequency & Duration:
    _____ 6 (Trial) Course of treatments

    _____ **Acute:** 2 to 3 treatments per week for 4 weeks

    _____ **Chronic:** 2 to 3 treatments per week for up to eight weeks and 1 to 2 treatment per week thereafter.

    _____ **Recurrent/Flare-Up** - 8 to 12 visits as needed over a 2 month period

    Medical Necessity:
    _____ As per AME report
    _____ Functional improvement is documented as defined in Section 9792.20 (e)
    _____ Pain with range of motion to above affected area
    _____ Decreased range of motion to above affected area

_____ See supporting documentation attached

If any additional information is required for your assessment please feel free to contact me at the numbers listed above. Otherwise if we do not receive a reply within the next five (5) working days we will assume we are authorized to provide the services as outlined per UR guidelines LC 4610 (g) (1).

Respectfully,

Dr.

_____

Authorized by: _____   Date:
_____

Authorization #: _____

Expert Witness Fees &
Acupuncture Expert Services Agreement

Litigation: $250.00 per hour for services including, but not limited to, review, research and analysis: reports, conferences, site visitation and survey where appropriate together with a review of all discovery materials and any other materials deemed necessary to reach and render an opinion in the subject litigation.

A minimum, non-refundable advance retainer fee of $2,000.00 is required. Initial work will be charged against the retainer. I am retained solely by the attorney/ attorney's firm (client) and no relationship exists between the attorney's client and me. The attorney/attorney firm is solely responsible for fee payment.

Deposition: Deposition fee will be $1000.00 to be pre paid by opposing counsel on or before the date of deposition.

Trial: $2,000.00 or a full eight (8) hours for trial appearance and testimony.

Cancellation: Counsel is required to provide forty-eight (48) hour notice of cancellation of scheduled testimony or be subject to a four (4) hour cancellation fee plus any travel expenses.

Travel: Client is responsible for travel arrangements and actual expenses. Travel fees are billed at $60.00 per hour. No fees will be advanced by this office.

Invoices: All invoices are due and payable within 15 (15) days of receipt. Invoices thirty (30) days past due will be charged interest at the rate of 1.5% per month (annual rate of 18%), and will be assessed a $200.00 late fee. Invoices sixty (60) days past due will be referred for collection and all legal remedies for payment pursued.

Payment: The attorney/attorney firm is solely responsible for fee payment.

Engagement: Your signature below indicates acceptance of this binding agreement and formal engagement of John Q. Acupuncturist, L.Ac. to provide expert witness services.

Authorized Signature / Title: _____

Date: _____

Sample Acupuncture Protocols

Legend:

Acupx=Acupuncture w/o stimulation.
EA=Electric Acupuncture
MFR=Myofascial release
HA=Headache
CS=Cervical Spine
TS=Thoracic Spine
LS=Lumbar Spine
VMO=Vastus medialis obliquus
TP=Trigger Point

Important to focus on dermatome distribution!

- Head (HA): Acupx Li 4 GB 21, UB10. MFR with ischemic compression to TP with preferred pain ointment.

- CS: EA TP in C3-C6 region. MFR with ischemic compression to TP with preferred pain ointment.

- TS: EA TP rhomboid musculature.T4-T12 region MFR with ischemic compression to TP with preferred pain ointment.

- LS: EA TP lumbar musculature. L4-S1 region MFR with ischemic compression to TP with preferred pain ointment.

- Shoulder (trapezius): EA TP trapezius region to include GB 21.MFR with ischemic compression to TP with preferred pain ointment.

- Shoulder (deltoids): EA TP deltoids to include LI 15. MFR with ischemic compression to TP with preferred pain ointment.

- Elbow: EA LI 10, LI 11, SJ 10, SI 8. MFR with stretch/counter stretch to triceps with preferred pain ointment.

- Wrist/Hand: EA (micro current) LI 4, Midway between H 7 & H 8, SI 8, LI 10. MFR with stretch/counter stretch to forearm TP with preferred pain ointment.

- Hip: EA GB 29, GB 30, UB 27, UB 53. MFR with ischemic compression to TP with preferred pain ointment.

- Knee: EA GB 34, K 10, SP 10, ST 34. Additional EA to VMO. MFR with ischemic compression to TP with preferred pain ointment.

- Ankle: EA GB 34, GB 40, K3, LV 4.

- Heel: EA GB 34, K3, UB 56, UB 57. MFR with ischemic compression to the gastrocnemius and soleus group with preferred pain ointment.

This is a short list of protocols to demonstrate the medical acupuncture approach to treatment.

Endnotes

[i] http://www.acupuncture.ca.gov/about_us/history.shtml
[ii] http://www.statefundca.com/about/History.asp

[iii] http://www.dir.ca.gov/dwc/SB863/SB863_Overview.htm
[iv] http://www.dir.ca.gov/dwc/WCGlossary.htm

www.ingramcontent.com/pod-product-compliance
Lightning Source LLC
Chambersburg PA
CBHW051820170526
45167CB00005B/2091